Practical
Pre-School

A-Z of Child Health

by Dr Neela Shabde Illustrated by Cathy Hughes

Contents

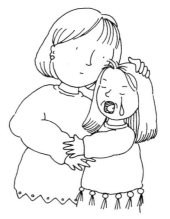

Published by Step Forward Publishing Limited
Park Court, Park Street, Leamington Spa CV32 4QN   Tel: 01926 420046
© Step Forward Publishing Limited 1999

A to Z of Child Health   ISBN: 1-902438-09 4

Introduction

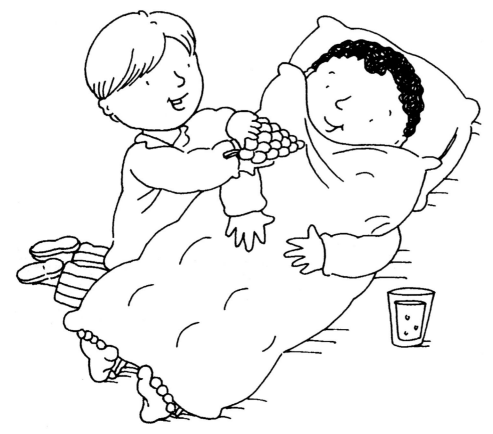

Caring for children puts an enormous responsibility on parents and carers. Healthy children will have healthy minds - enabling them to reach their potential in all areas of development.

Nurseries and pre-schools play an important role in providing an encouraging, stimulating and nurturing environment for children to learn about their world through play. Trained nursery staff can tell if a child is not reaching his or her developmental milestones. They also need to know how to detect acute symptoms of illness requiring urgent medical attention as well as chronic symptoms which affect a child's ability to get the most from their education.

Children in the early years are most vulnerable to catch infections as their immune system is maturing. However, children's health problems have a varied pattern and young children may be unable to describe their symptoms. The clinical picture can change rapidly and carers should be aware of the need for vigilance and the importance of seeking expert medical attention and advice whenever there is any doubt about a child's health.

The main aim of this book is to give clear information to anyone who is involved in caring for pre-school children, and to help them detect any significant symptoms and signs of common childhood illnesses so that appropriate action can be taken.

The list of conditions covered is not exhaustive and we have not covered congenital conditions or difficulties which could be classed as special educational needs. However, every attempt has been made to cover conditions which you are likely to come across in young children. A question and answer format is used to help you decide on the best course of action.

Dr Neela Shabde, consultant paediatrician (Community child health), North Tyneside Care NHS Trust.

Note: This book is not a medical text book neither does it aim to replace professional medical advice. It is a guide to some common childhood illnesses for information purposes only. It should not be used to replace professional advice. If you are in any doubt about a child's health or welfare then the proper professional services should be consulted.

First Aid and resuscitation

It is important that you know the basics of First Aid. Ideally, everyone on your staff should receive basic training to enable them to give the best possible First Aid treatment in an emergency. This is for your own peace of mind as well as to reassure the parents of the children in your care. Information about First Aid training in your area may be obtained from:

St John's Ambulance,
1 Grosvenor Crescent,
London SW1X 7EF
Tel: 0171 235 5231

St Andrew's Ambulance,
St Andrew's House,
48 Milton Street,
Glasgow G4 0HR
Tel: 0141 332 4031

There is no legal requirement for there to be a qualified First Aider in a nursery. However, the Health Education Guide recommends that a school has one nominated qualified First Aider who has undergone approved training for 18 hours. This is renewable every three years. The principles and practice of First Aid are included as part of the curriculum for NNEB students and most colleges offer a separate First Aid certificate however, this would need updating regularly.

British Red Cross Society - You will find local numbers in your telephone directory.

ABC check
You may have to deal with an emergency at any time, so familiarise yourself with the most important principle of First Aid - the ABC check:

Airway - is it clear?
Breathing - is the child breathing?
Circulation - is there a heart beat?

Airway - Lift the chin with two fingers and tilt the head back. If the child is breathing, place him in the recovery position.

Breathing - If the child is not breathing, start artificial ventilation.

Circulation - Check the child's pulse by pressing on the groove of the neck, in front of the large muscle at each side. If you cannot feel a pulse, then start cardio pulmonary resuscitation (CPR).

If the child is unconscious, ask someone to call an ambulance. While you wait the child should be put in the recovery position as follows:

The child lies on his side almost on the tummy with the arm underneath preventing him rolling forward. The head should be tilted back to keep the airway open.

In an unconscious baby tilt the head back slightly whilst holding the baby securely in your arms. This prevents them from inhaling his/her own vomit.

Recovery position

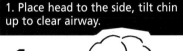
1. Place head to the side, tilt chin up to clear airway.

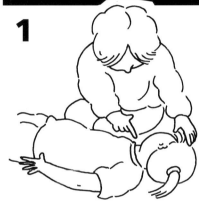

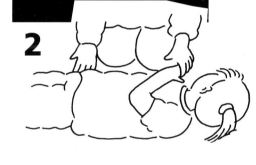
2. Tuck arm closest to you under child's bottom, palm up; bring the other arm over child's body.

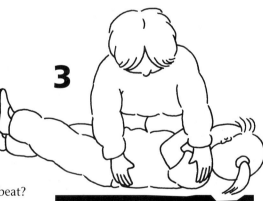
3. Hold on to child's shoulder and waist. Cross the child's legs - leg furthest away from you on top.

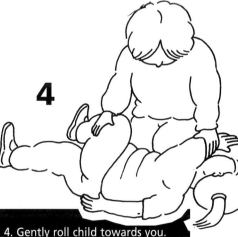
4. Gently roll child towards you. Bend knee of top leg up to support body. Place top arm palm down and release lower arm. REMEMBER to straighten airway.

Check your First Aid kit. It should contain:

+ **Cotton wool**
+ **Surgical tape**
+ **Sterile dressings**
+ **Absorbent wipes**
+ **Tweezers**
+ **Triangular bandages**
+ **Crepe bandages**
+ **Tubular finger bandages**
+ **Scissors**
+ **First Aid handbook**
+ **Safety pins**
+ **Non-adhesive absorbent dressing**
+ **Antiseptic wipes**
+ **Assorted waterproof plasters**

This can vary depending on your local authority regulations. Check with them first

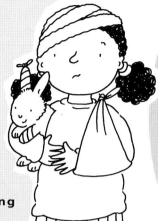

FIRST AID EMERGENCY SITUATIONS

1 Unconsciousness

2 Shock

3 Cessation of breathing and heart beating

4 Burns and scalds

5 Cuts, bruises and bleeding

6 Broken bones

7 Poisoning

8 Choking and suffocation

9 Joint and muscle injury

Resuscitation

If the child is not breathing, you should start artificial ventilation at once by breathing for him.

+ Tilt the child's head back slightly and lift the chin with two fingers of the other hand to open the airway. You may need to clear the airway.

+ Pinch nose shut with two fingers of one hand whilst supporting the child's jaw with the other hand.

+ After taking a deep breath, open your mouth wide and seal your lips over the child's mouth. Breathe into the child's mouth, taking a fresh breath yourself after each of the ventilations. If the procedure is correctly applied the child's chest will rise and then fall. If the child has a pulse then continue artificial ventilation at the rate of one breath every three seconds ie 20 breaths per minute until the child can breathe by himself. As soon as regular breathing is established, place the child in the recovery position.

Proceed to CPR if the child has no pulse in order to keep the vital organs supplied with oxygen as permanent brain damage can ensue after only three minutes without oxygen.

CPR is a technique which combines artificial ventilation to deliver air into the child's lungs and external heart massage through chest compressions to enable the oxygenated blood supply to reach the organs in the body.

+ Open airway and check breathing (as described above).

+ Give artificial ventilation (as described above).

+ Check for a pulse by placing your two fingers into a groove between the child's wind pipe and the large muscles in the neck, just below the jaw. Feel for five seconds. If there is no pulse then start chest compressions.

+ Place the child on a hard flat surface and find the breastbone (the bone that runs down the centre of the chest).

+ Place two fingers (middle and index finger) at the spot where the ribs meet and then place the heel of your hand over the lower half of the child's breastbone, keeping your fingers off the child's ribs.

+ Press down to a depth of 2.5 - 3.5 cm (1"-1.5") and then release the pressure

+ Do this five times within three seconds at a rate of 80-100 compressions per minute (counting the compressions 'one and two and three', and so on, as you do). Alternating with one breath of artificial ventilation continue, until the ambulance arrives.

It is important not to apply too much pressure or force as you can break the child's ribs.

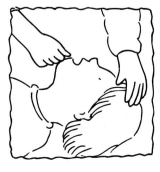

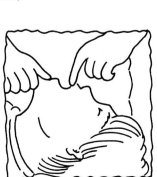

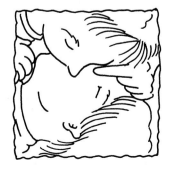

Policies and procedures

Professional childcarers have a responsibility to ensure that the health and welfare of the children in their care is paramount. Any facility registered under the Children Act 1989 needs to have a policy on health, safety and child protection, to make sure that everyone involved in the setting - staff, volunteers and parents - is clear about their responsibilities and the procedures to be followed, to promote a healthy safe environment and to protect the well-being of children and adults.

Legislation

Although the Children Act 1989 is the major piece of legislation covering providers of day care for children under eight years, other health and safety legislation has to be complied with.

▲ Health and Safety at Work Act 1974

▲ Health and Safety Regulations 1981

▲ Management of Health and Safety at Work Regulations 1992

▲ Electricity at Work Act 1989

▲ Fire Precautions Act 1971

▲ Food Safety Act 1990

▲ Reporting of Injuries, Diseases and Dangerous Occurrences Regulations 1985

▲ Disability Discrimination Act 1995

It is unlikely that you will have in-depth knowledge of any of this legislation, and you are not expected to. This is where your local authority under-eights department, which registers and inspects day care facilities, can give advice and help. Each local authority has its own regulations, procedures and systems for day care providers to follow, so the information in this book can only be a guide. You should check on local policies, procedures and proformas and with your own professional organisations.

Keeping records

Before admitting any child into your care, you should discuss with parents the stage of development their child is at; any health problems, allergies, disabilities, special dietary needs and the child's immunisation records. It is good practice to record all of this on the child's profile, together with the name, address and phone number of the

child's doctor, health visitor and emergency contact numbers for parents. In many areas parents are encouraged to share their child's health records with carers. To make sure that details are accurate at all times, it is essential that you ask for the information to be updated at regular intervals.

Make sure everyone knows where this information is kept and remember to take it with you if you take a child to hospital as the doctors will need to know details about immunisation and possible allergies, for example.

When children are unwell

If a child is unwell, they should not be in any care provision - not only to prevent the risk of infection spreading but also because constant nursing and attention may be needed. This policy should be made quite clear to all parents when their child starts with you. Persistent colds, coughs and other infections need to be discussed with parents and children should only be accepted again when they are fit enough. Periods of exclusion for communicable diseases should be obtained from your local health authority department of public health. In the case of vomiting and diarrhoea you should specify how long a child should be kept away - at least 24 hours after the condition has stopped and the child is fully fit.

If a child becomes unwell whilst in your care, it is your responsibility to ensure that the child's parents are informed. The child should be allowed to rest away from other children but within contact of an adult until collected by parents. When other children are exposed to communicable diseases and infections, all parents should be informed as soon as possible but always within 24 hours. This is important for all children but especially for those whose immune systems may be low. Confidentiality must be respected and the child who is unwell should not be named.

Administering Medicine

There is no legal duty which requires carers to administer medicine. Medication policies are recommended in all care facilities. Although a child on medication is best off at home, there may be occasions when a child can be re-admitted on doctor's advice but needs to complete a prescribed course of medicine. If you are offering a full day care service, you may be asked to help with this.

You may be asked to care for a child with special health needs, who perhaps is asthmatic or has a life-threatening allergy for which prescribed medicine/procedures must be used. Before accepting any such child into your care, check with your insurance company that you will be covered and advise your local under-eights officer. Discuss the child's health needs fully with their parents and draw up a protocol to be followed in the case of emergencies. Make sure that you have professional instruction in the administration of medical procedures such as epipens. Confirm whose responsibility it is to check the shelf life of any medication and get both parents to countersign any agreements reached with review dates built in.

In all circumstances parents should have given medicine prior to expecting you to administer it, so that the child has no proven allergic reaction. Parents must also complete a medical consent form which names the prescribed medicine, times and doses of medication to be administered. This should be completed by the carer as any medicine is given and, if you work in group care, get the entry countersigned by a colleague who witnessed it. Confidentiality should be respected and a separate proforma per child used. A new consent form for each course of medicine is needed. All medicines should be kept out of reach of children and refrigerated if necessary.

Accidents and First Aid

Everyone involved in caring for young children should carry out a daily risk assessment of the environment and playrooms in which they are working. Do not assume that someone else has already done this! By being vigilant you can minimise the risk of accidents happening to the children in your care.

Your registering authority will require at least one emergency First Aid box to be kept in a safe place where all staff know where it is and how to access it. The contents should be checked regularly and items replaced. It is especially important for childminders to ensure that the First Aid box you use for your childminding service is separate to that used for your own family. A suggested list of contents is given on page 4 but it is worth checking for local guidance.

A First Aid kit should always be taken on outings. Obtain permission in writing to take children out and adhere to the recommended adult/child ratios. If you are a childminder it is important to carry identification that you are a childcarer and an emergency contact number should you be involved in an accident. Advice should be sought through your local authority adviser or the National Childminding Association (for address, see page 30).

First Aid is exactly what it says - first aid. All group care facilities should have at least one trained First Aider on duty at all times, although all staff should be encouraged to undertake training. In some areas, childminders have to agree to undertake full First Aid training within the first year of registration and this practice should be endorsed. If you have not yet attended a First Aid course, contact your local branch of the Red Cross or St Johns Ambulance.

Parents should give written permission for First Aid to be administered and for medical help to be sought in case of emergencies. This should be included in the formal form filling before the child starts with you.

If an accident occurs, no matter how minor, you as the childcarer should complete an accident report form, ensure that the child's parent has been informed and has countersigned to acknowledge this. Confidentiality should be respected at all times so it is important that details cannot be seen by another parent, and if another child was involved that child is not named. A sample accident record form is given on page 32 but others can be obtained through professional organisations. These records should be available for your inspection officer to see. It is also a good idea to check with your local authority for any preferred proformas and the length of time records should be kept.

For more serious accidents, for example a broken limb, hospitalisation or the death of a child (or staff member) you have a duty to report this under the Reporting of Injuries, Diseases and Dangerous Occurrences Regulations to your local Health and Safety Executive. Advice on the procedures for this should be obtained from your own local authority department.

All children develop at different rates and part of the work of health professionals is to monitor the progress of each child as an individual within the accepted sequence of growth and development milestones. As a childcarer you can work in partnership with parents to reassure, or identify any potential problems and tactfully encourage them to seek appropriate help and guidance. Minor accidents are common in childhood and some can be linked with different stages of development whilst the child is exploring and making sense of the world around them. Usually accidents have a plausible explanation and although possibly could have been avoided are accepted as that.

Child protection

Occasionally, however, injuries are caused deliberately by adults who are responsible for their children - these are known as non-accidental injuries and are a form of child abuse. As a childcarer you have a responsibility to work with the local social services and police to protect children. Procedures to be followed will have been drawn up by the Local Area Child Protection Committee and you should familiarise yourself with their guidance.

Child protection is a complex subject and if you have not had any child protection training, ask your line manager, contact your local authority or the National Society for the Prevention of Cruelty to Children for advice or literature.

If you feel that something is not right with a child or a child discloses that they are being abused, remember that you are not alone. You are part of a professional network which will work together to help the child, and offer support to both the child and their family. If a child makes a verbal disclosure, you should overcome your own feelings, and reassure the child that it was right to tell you. Listen, but do not put words into the child's mouth and never promise that you will keep any information a secret. Tell the child that you will need to discuss anything you see or hear with your line manager or local social services duty desk. Keep a written record of events, making the report factual, including dates and times. Ensure that you know the routes of referral in operation in your area.

Protecting yourself

In order to be able to provide continuity of care for children, you need to ensure that you are fully fit. As a childcarer, discuss with your own doctor the immunisations that will protect you and if advised to have boosters or additional innoculations, take that advice! Rubella, tetanus, tuberculosis, polio and hepatitis are those that are usually recommended, but only you and your doctor know your own medical history and can make the right decisions.

Check that parents have used items such as teething gel, baby creams and sun protection cream on their child prior to using these yourself. Always use products supplied by parents - do not be tempted to use your own. If you work in a group care setting, follow the guidelines set down in your facilities procedures.

▲ Never administer anything without parents' written consent.

▲ Check your own insurance position.

▲ Ensure that you know the procedures and regulations of your registering authority.

▲ Remember to follow procedures and complete relevant paperwork at the right time.

▲ Make sure that you are up-to-date with current thinking and practice.

This will not only protect you but will ensure that you are giving a professional service.

Collecting evidence for childcare qualifications

If you are studying for childcare qualifications, such as an NVQ, you will need to build up a portfolio of evidence. This will be used by your assessor to check that you are competent as a childcare worker, and will be your underpinning of knowledge.

Evidence from past experience
(known as Accreditation of Prior Learning)
This will include any courses or talks which you have attended in recent years concerning the subject of child health. This could include:

▲ First Aid

▲ Child protection

▲ Food handling

▲ Child development

▲ The Diploma in Childcare Practice (run by the NCMA)

▲ Courses run by the PLA, such as IPP, DPP

▲ One-off talks, on such issues as ADHD and Aids

Evidence that you have attended the course or talk should be available, together with any notes or information obtained. It is quite useful to have a training record card where you can record what training you have attended.

Information relating to child health issues
Collect leaflets and read any books about the subject. Make brief notes and keep them in your portfolio, to show that you have read the book/leaflet and understand the significance to child health issues.

Work products
These can include:

▲ Leaflets or paperwork relating to child health issues which are given to parents within your setting.

▲ Daily diaries of your care of the children (listing nappy changes, meal times, and so on).

▲ Copies of menus provided for children in your care (particularly if there are special dietary needs).

▲ Copies of any accident reports completed by you.

▲ Records of medication given to children in your care, and the parental consent for this.

▲ Photographs, videotape recordings or audio tapes taken or made by you which show how you deal with health issues within your setting. This could include photographs or video footage of equipment and resources used in caring for the health of children in your care (although the assessor would probably wish to inspect the real thing).

▲ Records of any displays or project work which you have done within your setting relating to child health issues.

All work products should carry:

▲ Your name.

▲ The work setting in which they were produced.

▲ A countersignature to indicate that it is genuine (this can sometimes be a problem if you are working on your own, say as a childminder).

Confidentiality:
It is **very important** that you ensure that confidentiality is maintained. It must not be possible to identify any children or their families. It is always useful to obtain written permission from parents before you photograph or record their children. Always keep a copy of their permission.

Child observations and case studies
Any child observations which relate to the health of a child could be used.

A case study is a written account by you over a period of time. As well as observation details the case study could include details of a child's home situation and any agencies involved (such as speech therapist or health visitor). Also included should be details of any support which you give to the child and the family.

Again, it is very important that all materials are treated as confidential and that the child or family cannot be identified.

Policies and procedures of the setting
You must show that you have knowledge of the various policies and procedures relating to child health issues. This can be done by such methods as:

▲ Annual inspection reports (particularly useful for childminders, as they set their own policies and procedures).

▲ Staff induction. Have a copy of the group's policy document, with confirmation that you have read and understood it (with a countersignature of the person who carried out the induction).

▲ Details of hygiene procedures (dealing with spillages of bodily fluids, use of Latex gloves, and so on).

▲ A list of the contents of the First Aid box(es). Add notes as to why the items are included.

▲ Details of communicable diseases and exclusion times from the childcare setting.

Your own health
Have details of any relevant immunisation and injections you have had which will protect the children and the families with whom you work. This could include:

▲ Polio

▲ Rubella

▲ TB

▲ Hepatitis

To work in a childcare setting it is also necessary for you to complete a health declaration as part of the statutory checks. This could also be noted in your portfolio.

There are other methods of collecting evidence which will be used by an assessor, such as direct observation, questioning and inspection of the setting. However the evidence gathering suggestions mentioned above are ones which you can gradually prepare ready for the visit of your assessor.

This is not a complete list. The rules are:

▲ Include anything in your portfolio which you feel would be relevant.

▲ Never throw anything away!

▲ Record everything!

Information supplied by The Association of Advisers for the Under-Eights and their Families (AAUEF).

Accidents

Accidents are a significant problem in childhood. They are the most common cause of death in children over the age of one in Britain. Accidents also cause handicap and suffering to children and families. Some common accidents are covered in this book.

Children are curious and inquisitive by nature, they love to explore their environment without appreciating the risks and the dangers involved. Therefore, it is vital that adults caring for them ensure that the environment is relatively free from potential hazards.

A number of measures can be taken, such as restraining children in cars, which is essential to prevent death or serious injury in the event of an accident. You can also help children by teaching road safety as well as highlighting potential hazards in the playground and at home.

Most accidents are relatively minor. However, you and your staff should familiarise yourselves with the basic life saving First Aid techniques so that you are confident that you could respond appropriately in the event of a serious accident.

If the child is unconscious, check the following:

1 That the child is breathing and has a pulse. If they are, put them in the recovery position while you wait for the ambulance.

2 If the child is not breathing, start resuscitation immediately before attending to any other injury.

3 Whether there is severe bleeding which needs immediate treatment.

4 Whether there are other injuries - treat the injury you consider to be most serious.

The Child Accident Prevention Trust runs a series of seminars on different aspects of accident prevention including risk assessment, communication of child safety and how to compile an effective plan.

For further information contact:
Child Accident Prevention Trust,
Clerks Court,
18-20 Farringdon Lane,
London EC1R 3HA
Telephone: 0171 608 3828.

Anaphylaxis

Anaphylaxis is a rare but the most severe form of allergic reaction. It requires immediate medical attention or it can be fatal. It causes sudden constriction of the airway and a drop in blood pressure leading to collapse.

Common causes

+ Bee stings

+ Medicines - particularly those based on penicillin

+ Foods - peanuts, eggs, shell fish, cow's milk

Symptoms

Symptoms emerge a few minutes after the child has been in contact with the allergen. Initially they may experience an itching or burning feeling in the lips, mouth or throat. They may also develop:

+ a blotchy, itchy, raised rash

+ hives

+ pallor or sweating

+ swelling of lips, eyelids and tongue

+ anxiety

+ puffy face and neck

+ difficulty breathing

+ faintness, excessive drowsiness and loss of consciousness - collapse

Action

Call for an ambulance immediately. Whilst waiting, put the child in the recovery position (follow the basic First Aid). If a child has a known allergy and has been prescribed adrenalin it should be given without delay as advised (there should be a written protocol for that individual child).

The Anaphylaxis Campaign has produced a video, *Learning to live with Anaphylaxis*, which may be used for training. For details about this and any information on caring for children with anaphylaxis, contact:

The Anaphylaxis Campaign
PO Box 149
Fleet
Hampshire
GU13 9XU

Asthma

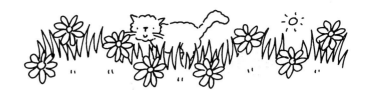

Asthma is a very common, chronic disease in children which affects the air passages. It is considered as an allergic response which may be triggered by a number of allergens for example, infection by a virus, house dust mite, pollen, animal hair, dander (animal dandruff), food, exercise, emotional stress, smoke. This leads to a narrowing of the tubes/air passages in the lungs (bronchi) as a result of inflammation of the lining of the air passages, contraction of the muscles within the walls lining the tubes and an increase in the secretion of mucus. This leads to difficulty in breathing/breathlessness and wheezing (which is a whistling noise coming from the chest).

It is important to recognise the symptoms of asthma because, if untreated, it may adversely affect the quality of life. It may also affect growth. A serious asthmatic attack can kill. Asthma may be accompanied by other conditions such as eczema or allergic rhinitis (inflammation of the lining of the nose) commonly known as hay fever and tends to cause symptoms in the spring and summer months. It often runs in families either in isolation or associated with other allergic conditions.

What are the symptoms?
A recurring dry cough may occur with a cold after exercise and sometimes only at night;
+ wheezing;
+ breathlessness;
+ tightness in the chest.

Depending on the severity of the attack, the following symptoms may be present:
+ difficulty in speaking
+ drowsiness
+ bluish discolouration of lips and tongue
+ vomiting
+ loss of appetite

Should you consult a doctor?
A severe attack needs immediate and urgent treatment. The child should be taken to the nearest accident and emergency department by calling an ambulance.
For less severe symptoms a consultation with the GP should be sought for an assessment and appropriate treatment.

What might the doctor do?
Assessment includes a detailed and thorough history of any possible allergens and other factors causing anxiety and distress such as bullying in school, difficulties at home and so on. The doctor may ask for a diary to be kept of symptoms and response to treatment for better long term management. In addition, in an older child, the severity of asthma may be assessed by using a peak flow meter which measures the capacity of lungs to exhale air. Sometimes a chest x-ray may be done if an infection is suspected or there is a poor response to the treatment.

What can be done to help
Asthma is managed by the child's parents/carers or in the case of an older child by himself. There is rightly a lot of emphasis on parent education so that the possible allergens may be avoided and the attack treated appropriately.

The drug treatment usually includes two types of drugs:
1 one for opening up the narrowed or constricted tubes in the lungs to ease breathing (a bronchodilator);

2 one for preventing attacks or reducing the frequency of attacks (corticosteroids - Becotide or Pulmicort).

The drug is usually inhaled and a number of devices are available. A doctor will prescribe the most appropriate one depending on the age of the child. Young children usually need a spacer (a large plastic tube which holds the drug whilst the child breathes in when ready). A face mask may be attached to the spacer for easier delivery of the drug in young children. In a severe attack only in very young children a nebuliser is used. This needs a pump to deliver the drug as a fine mist into a face mask.
Older children use a variety of inhalers for example aerosol inhaler or an inhaler which uses a powder form of drug.

Prevention
+ appropriate education of all concerned
+ avoid any known allergens
+ regular treatment to prevent further attacks or to reduce the severity of attacks
+ holistic approach to the treatment by supporting the child and the family during stressful situations.

If a child is known to have exercise induced asthma, he will benefit from taking the bronchodilator drug half an hour before their exercise schedule.

The National Asthma Campaign provides support for parents and carers of children suffering from asthma. An under-fives pack is available free from them at:

Providence House,
Providence Place,
London N1 0NT.

Telephone: 0171 226 2260.

They also have a Helpline (0345 010203) open Monday-Friday 9am-7pm.

Burns

Only First Aid for burns will be referred to here.
A burn is an injury to skin and deeper tissues following exposure to heat, fire, electricity or chemicals. In a superficial burn there may be first a reddened area or a blister, whilst in deeper burns layers of skin are affected which may leave a scar upon healing.

All burns apart from minor superficial burns will need treatment hospital as there may be:

+ risk of shock due to loss of fluid from the area of burn
+ risk of infection
+ risk of scarring

What should be done

1 In the first instance all burns should be cooled under running water for at least ten minutes. Do not delay in calling an ambulance if there are severe or extensive burns. For chemical burns, protect yourself from corrosive chemicals and put the affected area under cold running water for up to 20 minutes. Remove any contaminated clothing very carefully.

2 Cover the burned area with a clean, light, non-fluffy material, or with a bandage to prevent infection. Do not attempt to remove the clothing which has stuck to the burn.

3 Treat the child for shock if necessary as follows:
Lay the child down and raise the feet to a height of 20-30 cm (8-10 inches) on several pillows. Check and record pulse, breathing and consciousness level every ten minutes whilst waiting for the ambulance to arrive.

Don'ts
Do not use ointments or lotions on a burn
Do not break a blister
Do not use plasters or fluffy material to cover a burn

Signs of shock
Shock is due to a dangerous reduction of the amount of blood flowing to the other tissues. It inevitably causes reduction of oxygen to the tissues. It can result from bleeding either inside or outside the body, loss of fluids (dehydration) or a severe burn.

The signs are:
+ skin pale and grey
+ cold and clammy
+ rapid pulse becoming weaker
+ shallow and fast breathing
+ unusual restlessness
+ aggression
+ thirst
+ gasping for air
+ loss of consciousness

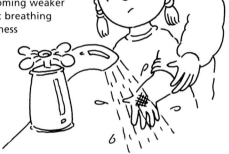

Chicken pox - also called varicella

This is one of the common, infectious diseases of childhood. It is usually a mild condition, showing itself with a characteristic itchy rash.

What are the symptoms?
The spots appear in crops every 3-4 days and develop quickly into blisters which leave a scab. They can appear all over the body including inside the mouth, anus, vagina or ears. They may leave scars if scratched too vigorously. Other symptoms may include mild fever, headache and severe cough in some cases.

What is the incubation period?
The incubation period is between 11-21 days. The child is infectious until all the spots are crusted. The number of cases is highest in late winter and spring.

What is the treatment?
There is no vaccine available against chicken pox. Treatment is mainly aimed at the symptoms of fever and itching. Calamine lotion on the spots will have a soothing effect. Sometimes antihistamines (anti-itching) may be needed. Itchiness may also be relieved by bathing the child in warm water containing a handful of bicarbonate of soda.

What is the outlook?
Children usually recover completely within 7-10 days after the onset of the symptoms.

An attack of chicken pox gives lifelong immunity from the disease. However, the virus remains dormant in the body and may cause shingles in later life.

Are their any complications?
Most commonly a secondary infection due to scratching. The child may develop pneumonia (infection of the lungs) and rarely inflammation of the brain, encephalitis.

Children with depressed immune systems are at greatest risk. This may be due to the child being on chemotherapy or taking oral cortico steroids.

An antibiotic will be required if there is secondary infection.

Cold sores

These are caused by a virus - a strain of herpes simplex virus. They are tiny blisters on and around the lips and the nostrils or anywhere on the face. The first attack usually presents as mouth ulcers. After the initial infection the virus usually lies dormant in the nerve endings which may be reactivated later to cause cold sores.

What are the symptoms?

+ The blisters may appear as a single blister or in clusters.

+ A tingling sensation around the mouth usually 4-12 hours before any blister appears.

+ Blisters which may be itchy and burst to form a crust and heal within a few days.

What can be done to help?

Usually no treatment is needed as they cause a minor inconvenience. If blisters recur frequently, a cream containing the anti-viral drug acyclovir may be used.

Cold sores are very contagious. To reduce the chance of spreading the virus, both to other children or other parts of the body, try to discourage the child from touching the blister or sucking their fingers. Also encourage frequent hand-washing. The child should avoid close bodily contact or kissing other children. They should use their own towel or face cloth. As cold sores can develop after exposure to the sun, use sun block cream on lips and nose.

What is the outlook?

There is no cure and the child may have recurrences throughout life but these become less frequent with time.

- -

Common cold (coryza)

The common cold is a virus infection of the nose and throat, which causes inflammation of the mucous membranes. It occurs very frequently in young children - up to five or six times a year. It may increase in frequency when a child starts to attend pre-school or nursery as they come across a number of viruses which can cause the common cold.

Symptoms

+ runny nose

+ sneezing

+ sore throat

+ cough

+ blocked nose

+ runny eyes

+ usually a fever

+ aches and pains in muscles

Cold viruses are spread in droplets which may be sneezed or coughed and are inhaled by others. They can also spread by direct contact.
Symptoms usually begin 1-3 days after infection.

Are there any complications?

It can cause bronchitis, bronchiolitis or pneumonia, which affects the lungs. Secondary bacterial infection may occur in the ears and/or sinuses. It can also trigger an asthma attack.

What can be done to help?

It usually takes a week to clear up. For symptomatic relief, keep the child warm but not so much as to increase their temperature. You could increase the moisture in the atmosphere by humidifying the air. Give the child plenty of fluids/drinks.

Paracetamol liquid may be given to relieve body ache and sore throat.*

Should you consult a doctor?

You should consult a doctor if the child is not drinking and their temperature is over 39°C (102°F), if the child is very unwell, if there is no improvement in cough in five days or symptoms are persisting after ten days.

The child may also need to be seen if they develop any other symptoms or any of the complications.

What is the outlook?

There is no way of preventing the common cold. To reduce risk of infection, avoid taking babies into crowded places. It is good manners for children to learn to cover the mouth when coughing but this does not necessarily prevent contamination. Very young children cannot manage to blow their own noses but you can help them. Use tissues which can be disposed of rather than handkerchiefs.

*See Administering medicine page 5

Conjunctivitis

Conjunctivitis is an inflammation of the thin, transparent membrane which lines inside the eyelids and covers the whites of the eyeballs.

How is it caused?
It may be caused by:
+ a viral infection
+ a bacterial infection
+ as a result of an allergy
+ a foreign body
+ chemicals

In the new-born baby, the infection may be transmitted by a mother who has chlamydial, gonorrhoeal or genital herpes infection. It may also result from the germs which are normally present in the birth canal.

What are the symptoms?
It may affect one or both eyes:
+ redness
+ sore eyes
+ itchiness and irritation of the eyes
+ clear thick yellowish discharge from the eyes leading to sticky eyelids - the child may be unable to open eyes in the morning (clear discharge usually indicates viral conjunctivitis whilst yellowish points to a bacterial infection)
+ swollen eyelids with clear discharge suggestive of allergic conjunctivitis

Is it serious?
It is a potentially serious condition in new-born babies, but with prompt treatment a child should recover completely.
In older children it is not serious but warrants appropriate action.

Should the doctor be consulted?
The doctor should always be consulted as soon as possible, particularly in babies.

In older children the doctor will assess for a foreign body and a serious disorder so that appropriate treatment may be given.

What might the doctor do?
The doctor will prescribe an antibiotic ointment or eye drops for a bacterial conjunctivitis and anti-inflammatory eye drops for viral conjunctivitis.
The child may need oral or intra venous antibiotics for a severe bacterial infection.
The child may be referred to an eye specialist if there is no improvement within a few days or if there is a suspicion of a foreign body.

What can you do to help?
+ The child's eyes should be gently bathed with cotton wool soaked and then squeezed out in cooled, boiled water, starting at the inner corner of the eye and wiped outwards.
+ Meticulous hand washing after touching the infected eye.
+ Keep the child's face-cloth and towels separate.
+ There is no need to exclude the child from nursery - as long as he is seen by the doctor and treatment commenced.

What is the outlook?
The new-born baby should recover completely if treatment is given promptly.
In older children the outlook is good. There is no serious risk to vision.

- -

Croup

Croup is usually caused by a viral infection. It causes inflammation and constriction of the upper airway leading to the lungs. It therefore results in a peculiar sound when the child breathes in and is called stridor. It usually occurs in young children between six months and three years but can affect older children. Younger children are more susceptible because of their narrower airways.

Croup is usually a mild, self-limiting illness but can frighten parents because of the symptoms of stridor and harsh barking cough. Occasionally it can cause severe breathing difficulties requiring emergency assessment and treatment.

What are the symptoms
It usually starts with a mild coryzal illness/common cold. After 24 - 48 hours:

+ croaking/barking cough

+ hoarse voice

+ noisy breathing

+ wheezing

In severe cases:

+ breathing difficulty, particularly when breathing in, and

+ bluish discolouration of lips and tongue indicating poor oxygen inhalation

In severe cases it is vital that you seek medical help at once

Action
In mild cases symptomatic treatment is indicated.
+ Keep the child calm.
+ Give paracetamol for fever and plenty of fluids.*
+ Keep the air in the child's room moist by boiling a kettle in the room, putting a wet towel in front of the radiator or using an air humidifier.

What might the doctor do?
The doctor will assess the severity of the croup and arrange further treatment.

In severe cases the child will be admitted to hospital. The child may be given oxygen and medicated inhalations.
In some cases the child may need help with breathing and will require a tube inserted through his nose or mouth into the windpipe until the inflammation settles. This usually takes a few days.

*See *Administering medicine* page 5

Diabetes mellitus

Diabetes is an uncommon condition which results because of the deficiency of a hormone called insulin, secreted by the pancreas gland.

Insulin is responsible for the normal metabolism of the sugar, glucose. In diabetes the glucose builds up in the blood and there is a disturbance of the body's chemical processes. There is defective absorption and storage of glucose in the body. The glucose builds in the blood and the unused glucose is passed out in large quantities of urine. Less energy is available to the body. As a result fats and proteins break down as an alternative energy source. This causes weight loss and produces poisonous waste products such as acetone and ketones.

Diabetes may be inherited. Its first presentation can be triggered off by a viral infection or for no apparent reason. Diabetic patients are extremely prone to infections.

What are the symptoms?
The increased levels of glucose in the blood (hyperglycaemia) cause:

+ frequent urination (can lead to bedwetting)
+ increased/excessive thirst
+ weight loss
+ lethargy and tiredness

In severe cases the child may present with:

+ vomiting
+ abdominal/tummy pains
+ drowsiness and confusion
+ dehydration

Without treatment the child may go into coma, which can be fatal.

What is the treatment?
If it is suspected that a child may have diabetes mellitus, the doctor should be consulted at once. Further tests will be arranged to confirm the diagnosis and treatment will be instituted usually in the hospital under the care of a paediatrician. The child and parents will be taught how to administer insulin and given advice about the diet. The emphasis is on the education of parents and older children about the condition so that diabetes can be successfully managed at home and in the community. The parents will be advised how to test for glucose in the urine and in the blood to enable them to adjust the dose of insulin to keep blood glucose levels normal. The blood glucose levels may fall too low causing a hypoglycaemic attack. The symptoms of a hypoglycaemic attack are:

+ dizziness or fainting
+ tummy pains
+ sweating and/or confusion

If the child develops any of these symptoms, give them a sweet drink or sweet food such as a biscuit or chocolate. Further symptoms may be drowsiness and loss of consciousness if a child is unable to eat or drink. They will then need an injection of Glucagon which will bring the blood sugar to a normal level.
It is advisable for the child to wear a bracelet and a medallion engraved with the details of their condition in case there are problems when the child is not with their parents.

Are there any complications?
Complications do not develop until 10-15 years after the onset. Poorly controlled diabetes can affect the heart and circulation, the kidneys, the eyes and the nervous system.

What is the outlook
Children with well-controlled diabetes should lead a normal life and should reduce the chances of complications. They will, however, need daily injections of insulin and monitoring of blood glucose and medical follow-up for life.

● ●

Diarrhoea

Diarrhoea is the passage of loose, watery bowel motions more frequently than normal. It is a serious symptom if the child is under one year of age. It may be accompanied by vomiting, fever and lead to dehydration due to profound water loss. Dehydration can be recognised by the following signs:

In young babies:
+ dry mucous membranes; tongue and oral mucosa
+ sunken eyes
+ sunken fontanelle (soft part of the top of the head)
in young children usually under one year
+ loss of skin turgor
+ passage of small amounts of concentrated urine
+ change in level of consciousness - drowsiness or irritability

In older children:
+ vomiting lasting for 12 hours
+ abdominal pains
+ dry mucus membranes - dry tongue and oral mucosa
+ sunken eyes

+ reduced or no urine output for more than six
hours during the day
+ reduced or no fluid intake for six hours

In most cases diarrhoea is not serious provided the child is drinking and passing water, and there is no vomiting. However, a child with diarrhoea should not be left in your care. If symptoms occur while a child is in nursery or pre-school, you should inform the parents or carers.

Possible causes of diarrhoea
In children under one year:
+ infection - gastro-enteritis or a response to other infection
+ food poisoning
+ side effects of medicines - mainly antibiotics
+ constipation with overflow incontinence

In older children:
+ infection (gastro-enteritis)

+ food intolerance
+ food poisoning
+ toddler's diarrhoea
+ side effects of antibiotics
+ excitement or emotional response

What can be done to help?

The main objective is to prevent dehydration by giving the child extra fluids. In children under one year, a special rehydrating solution is usually prescribed. The fluids should be offered in small amounts every two to three hours.

In older children, extra fluids should be given to prevent dehydration. Rehydrating solution can be given. All children should drink between 1-1.5 litres of fluids per day.

Should you consult a doctor?

If diarrhoea persists or there are other symptoms and signs, the child's doctor should be consulted for a further assessment.

Other possible causes of diarrhoea are:

Appendicitis - the child has a central abdominal pain which moves to the lower right side of the abdomen. It may be associated with vomiting. Consult a doctor immediately.

Intussusception - the young child has severe abdominal cramps with episodes of going pale and limp. The child may pass blood and mucus in stools resembling redcurrant jelly. You should consult a doctor immediately.

Coeliac disease - the child fails to thrive and the stools may be pale, bulky and foul smelling and difficult to flush. The child needs further assessment.

Eczema

Eczema is a common skin condition in children, often atopic (where the cause is not known). It causes a very itchy, dry, scaly rash. About 1 in 30 children develops atopic eczema. There is usually a strong family history of allergic disorder such as asthma, hay fever, rhinitis. It usually develops when the child is about two to three months old and the rash often disappears before the child reaches four. In some children the rash may appear between the ages of four to ten years.

Atopic eczema may be triggered:
+ when solid foods are introduced to a baby, particularly dairy products, eggs, wheat
+ by pet fur, wool or washing powders and fabric conditioners
+ by emotional stress

What are the symptoms?
+ Itchy, dry, red scaly skin with raised spots resembling pimples or minute blisters, which may be mildly weepy, affecting the scalp, face, neck, trunk, nappy area in babies, creases of arms and legs. It may also affect any part of the body.
+ In older children itchy, dry, scaly patches with broken skin which can get secondary infection. Most commonly affected areas are the face, neck, inside of elbows, wrists, backs of knees and ankles.
+ Thickening of skin in affected areas over a period of time
+ Extreme itchiness leading to sleeplessness

Are there any complications?
+ Secondary infection of skin with bacteria which can be very distressing.
+ Rarely secondary infection with herpes simplex virus causing widespread rash, high fever and enlarged lymph nodes.

What is the treatment?
+ The treatment consists of a cream to keep the skin moisturised and prevent it from drying out and cracking.
+ The child may be prescribed an anti-inflammatory skin cream with a weak steroid to reduce inflammation and itchiness.
+ They may be advised to avoid allergens such as dairy products, eggs or wheat as possible trigger factors.
+ The child may also be given an antihistamine medication to reduce itchiness and this will also help them sleep.
+ An antibiotic medicine/cream may be needed if the rash is infected.
+ The child may be sent to hospital for more intensive treatment with an intravenous antiviral drug if they develop secondary herpes simplex infection (eczema herpeticum).
+ Soap in the bath should be avoided. Make sure children dry their arms properly after playing in the water tray.

What is the outlook?
Most children grow out of eczema by the time they reach adolescence. The rash becomes less extensive as the child gets older. A very high percentage (up to 50 per cent) develop other allergic conditions, usually asthma.

Epilepsy

Recurrent fits or seizures are called epilepsy. Epilepsy occurs in about 1 in 200 children. It results from the disturbance of the electrical activity of the brain and may take different forms. The most common type is grand mal epilepsy affecting three quarters of children with epilepsy.

What are the symptoms?
Grand mal epilepsy
+ The child may show signs of irritability or behave unusually for a few minutes before the fit. The child then becomes rigid for a few seconds and usually falls to the floor unconscious.
+ There are jerky movements of all four limbs in a rhythmical manner with twitching of the face and rolling up of eyes lasting for a few seconds to a few minutes. The child clenches their teeth during which they may bite their tongue.
+ This is associated with the loss of consciousness, irregular breathing. The child's lips may turn blue. There may be incontinence of urine or bowel motions.
+ Following the fit, the child often becomes very quiet, confused and disorientated. The child may get a headache and sleep afterwards.

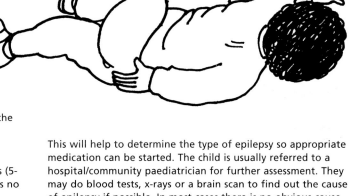

Petit mal epilepsy (Absence seizure)
The child stares into space ('daydreams') for a few seconds (5-10 seconds) and is unaware of their surroundings. There is no obvious convulsion. A number of petit mal seizures in succession can affect the child's school performance particularly and their normal activities. This form of epilepsy is often not recognised.

There are other less common forms of epilepsy such as benign focal epilepsy and complex partial seizures.
More commonly children under the age of six years get febrile convulsions (see page 16).

What can be done to help?
If a child has a grand mal seizure:
+ Place them in the recovery position and stay until the convulsion has stopped. Do not try to put anything in their mouth or hold their teeth apart.
+ Prevent them from injury during the fit.
+ Do not slap or shake a child in an attempt to stop the fit.
+ Remain calm.
+ Observe the child's fit carefully so that you can give an accurate history to their parent who can then describe it to the doctor. This will help in making a diagnosis.

What should you do?
+ You should inform the child's parents immediately and advise them to consult their doctor or take the child to the nearest accident and emergency department as soon as possible after the convulsion if the child has never had a grand mal convulsion.
+ If the child's convulsion is prolonged and the child remains unconscious for more than ten minutes call for an ambulance.
+ The parent should consult their doctor if the child has had less serious types of seizures.
+ Their doctor should be notified of any further seizures so that appropriate advice can be given.

What might the doctor do?
The doctor will take a detailed history of the child's behaviour and fits in order to establish a diagnosis and then arrange an EEG - electro encephalogram (brain wave activity).

This will help to determine the type of epilepsy so appropriate medication can be started. The child is usually referred to a hospital/community paediatrician for further assessment. They may do blood tests, x-rays or a brain scan to find out the cause of epilepsy if possible. In most cases there is no obvious cause (idiopathic epilepsy).
They may help the parents to identify the trigger factors such as flashing of lights, sitting too close to the television screen or computer.

What is the treatment?
Regular anticonvulsant drug therapy for a period of two to three years after the last seizure. It is then discontinued very gradually over several weeks.
In some cases, if a structural abnormality is causing seizures, surgery may be considered. The parents will be given information on epilepsy and how to manage it and they will advise you on what care should be taken in the nursery. You should make sure that everyone who works in the nursery - including helpers - knows of the child's condition, how to recognise the symptoms of a seizure and what to do.
Treat the child as normally as possible. Explain to their friends that they have epilepsy so that they will not be shocked or frightened if they have a seizure.

What is the outlook?
The outlook is variable and depends on the type of epilepsy. Most children (over three quarters) with grand mal epilepsy successfully treated with an anticonvulsant drug therapy do not have a recurrence.
Children with petit mal epilepsy with no educational problems do well without many problems.
Most children with benign focal epilepsy usually grow out of it by the time they reach puberty.

Febrile convulsions

A febrile convulsion is a fit or seizure associated with high temperature, usually over 39°C (102°F). The fever is usually a sign that there is an infection - viral or bacterial - in the body. It also results because of the rapid rise in body temperature.

Who does it affect?
It usually happens in children aged between six months and five years. It is quite common - about one in 30 will have had one by the age of five.

What is a convulsion?
It is caused by a storm of electrical activity of the brain. The child usually loses consciousness, becomes rigid and there is twitching and jerking of the limbs and the face, and rolling of the eyes. The breathing may become shallow and even stop for a few seconds to minutes, leading to change in colour. He may pass urine or faeces. The child then regains consciousness but may fall asleep or be drowsy and confused.

It is an extremely frightening experience. Most parents and carers fear the worst and think the child is dead or dying. However, febrile convulsions are not as serious as they look.

Should you consult a doctor?
If the fit lasts more than five minutes (it feels like hours!) you should call an ambulance. If this is a first fit which stops on its own, you should always tell the parents to consult their doctor.

What can be done to help?
With the first sign of a raised temperature it is important to keep the child cool but not over zealously. The following measures will help you to keep the child's temperature down:

+ Make sure that the child is not wearing too many clothes. Strip him down to vest and nappy/pants.

+ Give paracetamol in recommended dose depending on the child's age and weight every 4-6 hours*

Up to 1 year old - 120mg - (one 5ml medicine spoonful)
1 to 3 years old - 240mg - (two 5ml medicine spoonfuls)
4 years and over - 360mg - (three 5ml medicine spoonfuls)

+ Keep the temperature of the room down to 15°C (60°F) by switching the fire off and turning the heating down. You may use a fan.

+ Sponge the child's forehead, palms and soles with lukewarm water.

In the event of a fit what can you do?
Keep the child in the recovery position and follow the guidance above to reduce the child's temperature. This will help to prevent a further seizure.

What might the doctor do?
If this is a first fit the doctor will usually send the child to the hospital to be admitted for further assessment and observation. Treatment will be offered depending on the cause. The parents will be given advice on how to keep temperature down and to prevent and deal with future episodes. Where there have been recurrent fits rarely the child may be prescribed an anti-convulsant drug, diazepam, which is given into the child's back passage (rectum).

What is the outlook?
Although it is extremely frightening, a convulsion is not life-threatening. The child must be placed in the recovery position during a convulsion to prevent them inhaling body fluids into the lungs.

About a third of children will have a second attack with risk being highest in the first 24 hours. Children older than five years usually do not have febrile fits. A small number may later develop epilepsy.

- -

Fever

Fever is a temperature of 38°C (100°F) or over. It is usually a symptom that all is not well. It may be due to a viral or bacterial infection. It does not reflect the seriousness of the illness. However, in children usually in the first few months of life, it should be taken seriously. The rapid rise of temperature in children between six months and five years may cause a fit or convulsion (febrile convulsion).

There are many causes of fever. They also vary in young children and older children. Other associated symptoms may give a clue. Danger signs are:

+ temperature over 39°C (102°F)

+ abnormal rapid breathing or difficulty in breathing

+ drowsiness

+ irritability

+ non-blanching rash

+ vomiting

+ refusal to drink

What can you do?

+ Take the child's temperature and, if high, take measures to reduce it.

+ Give the child plenty of fluids to drink.

Should you consult a doctor?

+ If the child is a few months old.

+ If the child has a convulsion.

+ If there are any other worrying symptoms as mentioned above, the child's doctor should be consulted.

What might the doctor do?

The doctor will carry out an examination and treat the underlying cause of fever as appropriate. Further tests may be required in hospital.

What is the outcome?

The outcome depends on the cause of the temperature.

*See *Administering medicine* page 5

Gastro-enteritis

This is an inflammation of the stomach and intestines and results in diarrhoea and/or vomiting. It can also cause nausea, abdominal cramps and loss of appetite. It is common in children. It is usually a mild illness but can be serious in children under one year.

Most commonly it is a result of an infection with viruses. In children, one of the common causes is rotavirus. It may be caused by bacteria transmitted in foods or drinks, or through the air and by contact with infected faeces. It may also be a symptom of a generalised infection when the spread of the infecting organism to the bowel is through the blood stream. When it is caused by a parasite it is called dysentery.

It is difficult to prevent gastro-enteritis caused by a virus. However, the spread may be prevented by meticulous hygiene and taking great care to sterilise feeding equipment. It is important to store food at correct temperatures to prevent bacteria growing.

What are the symptoms?
The symptoms may appear 1-5 days after infection. These are
+ loose, watery stools/diarrhoea
+ vomiting
+ nausea
+ loss of appetite
+ abdominal pains/cramps
+ lethargy
+ fever

Is it serious?
It may be serious if the child becomes dehydrated as a result of fluid loss. Particularly in babies and young children, it is important for parents to consult their doctor as soon as possible. In older children the doctor should be consulted at once if, after six hours, treatment with clear fluids has failed to bring it under control.

Should the child be excluded from nursery?
It is desirable and reasonable to exclude the child until the acute attack is over and his stools or faeces return to normal. The child may attend nursery once he has stopped vomiting and if extra care is taken with personal hygiene such as hand washing, disposal of nappies, and so on.

What can be done to help?
+ You should stop all foods and milk as well as milk products.

+ Give plenty of clear fluids in small amounts frequently.

+ It is vital that the child is given plenty of fluids to replace fluid lost through diarrhoea and vomiting.

+ It is very important to maintain good hygiene with meticulous hand washing by the child, if old enough, and the carers.

+ Sterilise all feeding equipment with great care if the child is bottle fed.

What might the doctor do?
The doctor may prescribe a powder (oral rehydration powder which contains glucose and essential minerals) to be added to all the child's drinks. The child may be admitted to hospital if he is dehydrated and may need intravenous fluids. Once diarrhoea and vomiting are under control oral fluids are re-introduced gradually followed by a normal diet.

German measles (also known as rubella)

This is a mild, infectious disease caused by a virus. It may cause a rash, mild fever and swollen lymph nodes. In about a quarter of cases there is no rash and so it often goes unnoticed. Hopefully, the high immunisation uptake in the UK means that German measles is becoming rarer. The main risk of the illness is to the unimmunised pregnant woman. It is known to cause birth defects, blindness and deafness in the baby.

What are the symptoms?
+ Slightly raised temperature or mild fever.
+ Swollen lymph nodes in the neck and behind the ears. Other lymph nodes may be affected in a baby.
+ A rash consisting of tiny, flat pink/red spots starting on the face and spreading rapidly to the trunk and limbs, spots merging into each other causing a diffuse rash.
+ The rash is non-itchy on the second or third day and disappears within 3-4 days.
+ Some children may complain of joint pains.
+ Rarely there is an inflammation of the brain (encephalitis) and very low platelets (thrombocytopenia), which affects blood clotting.

What is the incubation period?
14 - 21 days

Is it serious?
It is not a serious illness in children. The greatest risk is to the unborn child.

Should the child be excluded from nursery?
Yes. German measles is infectious from one week before until four days after the rash appears. The child should be excluded from nursery for five days after the rash appears. Anyone who is pregnant and may have come into contact with the child should be informed.

Should you consult a doctor?
You should consult the doctor on the telephone and ask for the child to be seen if there are symptoms such as joint pain, stiff neck or headache.

What might the doctor do?
There is no specific treatment for rubella.

What can be done to help?
+ Give paracetamol to keep temperature down and give plenty of fluids.*
+ Avoid taking the child to public places and prevent him coming into contact with a pregnant woman.
+ Ensure that all children receive routine recommended immunisations.

What is the outcome?
Complete recovery within 7-10 days.
After a single attack - usually lifelong immunity.

*See *Administering medicine* page 5

Hand, foot and mouth disease

As the name suggests, this disease causes blisters in the mouth, on the backs of the hands and/or the feet. It is a mild viral infection and commonly affects children under the age of four. It is more common during the summer and early autumn.

What are the symptoms?
The incubation period is between 4-5 days.
✚ Mild fever.
✚ Blisters and/or ulcers in the mouth followed by blisters on the hands, and on the feet 1-2 days later. More commonly on the backs of hands and on the top surface of the feet.
✚ Malaise and frequently a sore throat.
✚ Not keen to eat.

What is the treatment?
There is no specific treatment available. It is supportive. Encourage the child to drink plenty of fluids. Paracetamol may be given to relieve pain and fever.*

What is the outlook?
Blisters in the mouth may last for 3-4 weeks whilst blisters on the hands and feet usually last for 3-4 days.

Should the child be excluded from nursery?
There is no need to exclude the child from the nursery. The disease poses an ordinary acceptable risk, such as that presented by the common cold or any other viral infection. The benefits of excluding a child do not outweigh the risks.

*See *Administering medicine* page 5

Head lice

Infestation with head lice is not uncommon in nursery and school age children as they can catch insects through direct contact, by sharing hats or combs. Head lice are very tiny, flat insects which survive on the human hair and suck blood. Head lice lay eggs, also called nits, at the root of the hair. These eggs are firmly attached to the hairshaft in contrast to dandruff which flakes off easily if the scalp is scratched. Head lice tend to prefer clean hair.

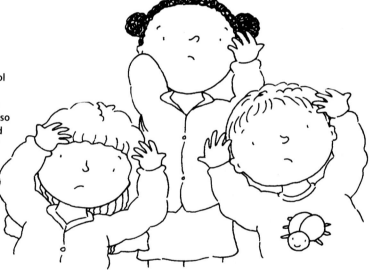

What are the symptoms?
✚ intense itching of the scalp
✚ tiny red spots on the scalp
✚ eggs which are whiteish and oval in shape seen on the hair near the bases

Is it serious?
No, it can be treated and the lice eradicated.

What can you do to help?
If you suspect that a child may be infested with head lice, examine the hair very carefully. You can use a very fine comb to run through the child's wet hair. You will be able to see the eggs as well as tiny crawling lice if you comb the child's hair over a piece of white paper. You should also check other children in the group.

Who should you tell?
Tell the child's parents and all other parents so they can be vigilant.

Should you consult a doctor?
Parents can treat head lice. However, if they are unsure or if their child has allergies or a skin condition they should consult their doctor. Similarly, if the treatment has not worked they should ask for a doctor's or the practice nurse's advice.

How can head lice be treated?
Special shampoo or lotion can be bought from a chemist. There will be instructions for use with the preparation. Some need a single application, others need to be used over a number of days.

Instructions should be followed carefully. All combs and brushes should be washed in boiling water. Other members of the group should be checked and treated. This will prevent the child being re-infected. Usually, one treatment is sufficient to get rid of head lice. Children's hair should be carefully combed with a fine tooth comb. Parents who prefer not to use chemical treatment may find that repeated combing through hair washed and treated with conditioner can be just as effective.

Should the child be excluded from nursery?
Yes, until after they have received treatment.

How can head lice be avoided?
Children should avoid sharing hats, combs and brushes with friends or family members. In the event of an outbreak, head lice repellents may be bought at the chemist.

Headaches

Headaches are not uncommon in older children and adolescents. One in five children may suffer from recurrent headaches. In very young children, however, headache is unusual. Headaches may accompany acute infections with fever, for example upper respiratory tract infection, sinusitis. It may also accompany toothache.

When should you take them seriously?
+ If they are severe, persistent or recurrent.
+ If there are other associated symptoms, for example vomiting, drowsiness, intolerance of bright light or stiff neck, immediate medical advice is needed.
+ Headache may also follow a very recent head injury. Immediate medical attention should be sought.
+ Headache may accompany abdominal pains. If recurrent and persistent you should consult the doctor.

What can be done to help?
If the child has no other symptoms and is generally well, you may give them an appropriate dose of paracetamol* and a drink. Let

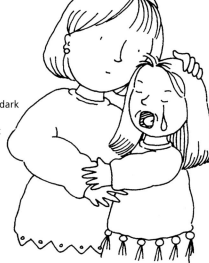

them lie down in a cool, dark room. If the child is hungry, give them a light snack. However, if the child seems unwell, or develops any other symptoms, contact the child's parents and tell them to consult a doctor at once.

What might the doctor do?
The doctor will take a detailed history and examine the child to try and determine the cause of the headache and any other symptoms. Further tests may be required depending on the findings.

*See *Administering medicine* page 5

Head injury

Minor knocks and bangs to the head are common in childhood. In most cases they are not serious and the child is back to their normal self in 10-15 minutes of the accident. In some cases a minor cut on the scalp or forehead can cause severe bleeding and it can be alarming.

Is it serious?
If there are other symptoms, such as drowsiness, lapses of unconsciousness or vomiting, you must seek medical attention immediately. The main risk of a head injury is shaking injury to the brain and bleeding inside the skull, which can cause brain damage. In rare cases it can be fatal.

What are the symptoms?
In cases of a minor head injury:
+ there may be no symptoms
+ a slight headache and/or a local swelling at the site of the injury.If there has been a significant blow to the head it may lead to concussion a brief period of unconsciousness usually lasting for a few seconds. This is a result of the brain being shaken inside the skull.
Common symptoms following concussion are:
+ confusion
+ period of unconsciousness
+ inability to remember events that happened just before the injury
+ blurring of vision
+ dizziness
+ drowsiness
+ irritability
+ vomiting
+ discharge of blood or straw coloured fluid from the nose or ears - this indicates that there may be a skull fracture.
In more severe cases, the period of unconsciousness may last for a few minutes or the child may even go into a coma. It is important to remember that symptoms of concussion may not appear for several hours.

Should you consult a doctor?
You should consult a doctor immediately or take the child to the nearest accident and emergency department at the hospital if there

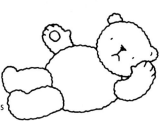

are the following symptoms:
+ unconsciousness even for only a few seconds
+ confusion and abnormal drowsiness
+ persistent vomiting
+ blood or straw coloured fluid leaking from the nose or the ears
+ laceration or cut on the head requiring further treatment
+ If you have any concerns regarding the child's behaviour even hours after the injury, for example pallor, unusually quiet and drowsy, no interest in food.

What might the doctor do?
A careful and thorough medical examination will be carried out. If there is a scalp wound, it may need to be stitched.
An x-ray of the skull may be taken if a fracture is suspected. A CT scan may be performed, which may show signs of bleeding in the brain. An emergency operation by a neurosurgeon may be needed to stop the bleeding and remove a clot. If there is a fracture of the skull pressing on the brain this will also need an operation in a neurosurgical unit.
A child with significant head injuries will need to be observed in hospital for at least 24 hours after the injury for further assessment so that appropriate treatment is carried out.

What can be done to help?
+ If a child has a head injury and you are not sure how serious it is, you should get them checked by a doctor at the accident and emergency department at the hospital.
+ If the child complains of a headache but is otherwise well, you can observe them for a few hours. However, if they develop any abnormal symptoms, as mentioned above, you must consult the doctor immediately.
+ If there is a wound on the scalp which is bleeding, press a clean cloth or a pad on it for at least 5-10 minutes until the bleeding stops.

What is the outlook?
Usually there should be no long-term effects of minor head injuries. However, severe head injury may cause permanent brain damage leading to a physical and/or mental disability.

Immunisation

The following is the recommended immunisation schedule in Britain.

Every child has a right to protection from infectious diseases. This is best achieved by ensuring that children are offered all immunisations they are entitled to - you can play an important role by encouraging parents to seek appropriate medical advice for their children's immunisation queries.

Vaccine	Age	Notes
Diphtheria/ Tetanus/Pertussis (D/T/P); Hib; and Polio	1st dose 2 months 2nd dose 3 months 3rd dose 4 months	Primary course
Measles/mumps/rubella (MMR)	12-15 months	Can be given at any age over 12 months
Booster D/T and polio, MMR second dose	3-5 years	Three years after completion of primary course
BCG	10-14 years or infancy	
Booster tetanus diphtheria and polio	13-18 years	

Children should therefore have received the following vaccines:

By 6 months:	3 doses of D/T/P, Hib and polio
By 15 months:	measles/mumps/rubella
By school entry:	4th D/T and polio; second dose measles/mumps/rubella
Between 10 and 14 years:	BCG
Before leaving school:	5th polio and T/D

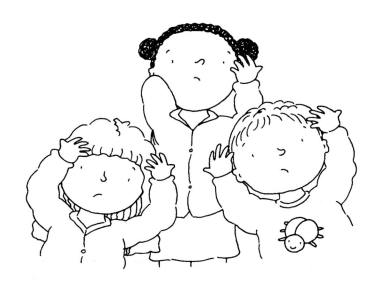

Impetigo

Impetigo is a common, highly infectious, skin condition caused by a bacterial organism known as staphylococcus. The organism is normally carried in the nose and on the skin. It most commonly affects the nose area around the mouth though it may affect any other part of the body in school-age children. It is also known to affect babies, especially the nappy area. The conditions such as eczema, scabies or where the skin is broken may pre-dispose to impetigo as the organism can enter and infect the skin.

Is it serious?
It is usually not serious but it is highly contagious and therefore needs to be treated promptly.

Will the child need to be excluded from nursery?
Yes, the child should be kept away from nursery or school until they have been treated and the infection has completely cleared up. It usually takes about 5 days.

What are the symptoms?
It starts as small blisters around the nose or the mouth. The blisters burst and then ooze. These moist blisters gradually enlarge and harden to form straw/yellowish coloured crusts and scabs. They are usually not painful but they can be slightly itchy. If not treated it may last for weeks to months.

What should you do first?
If you suspect impetigo, ask the parent to arrange to take the child to the doctor for treatment as soon as possible. Discourage the child from touching the sores and therefore from spreading the infection to other areas. Keep the child's face cloth and towel separate.

What might the doctor do?
The doctor may prescribe a local antibiotic cream/ointment or an oral antibiotic depending on the extent of the infection.

What can be done to help?
Before applying the cream/ointment, remove the crusts gently by washing with warm water and pat dry with a gauze or a soft paper towel. Keep the child's face cloth/towel and any bedding separate. Keep the child's fingernails short to reduce the risk of spreading the infection to other parts of the body. Once treated, keep the area well moisturised with emollient cream to prevent skin breaking.

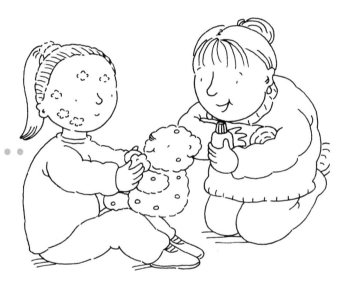

Itchiness

Itchiness is a symptom of underlying skin problems. It may affect a part of the body or the whole body. It may be due to a number of causes from allergic reaction to infection or an infestation by parasites. Rarely nervous tension and worry can also cause itching. Itching can be distressing and scratching can cause infection. It is important to receive prompt treatment of the underlying cause.

What are the common causes?
+ Eczema, allergic reaction to food or drug or skin contact with an irritant leading to hives.
+ Infection/infectious disease - chicken pox, scabies, fleas, ringworm.

Is it serious?
It is rarely serious but it should be promptly treated.

What should you do first?
You can check for the common causes depending on the site of itching. For example, itchiness in the hair may be due to ringworm, on the feet could be due to athlete's foot, itching around genitals and anus could be due to worms or thrush and in between fingers could be due to scabies. You can check for contact with pet - fleas which may be the cause. Check if the child has ingested any new food or has come into contact with anything unusual.
You may apply calamine lotion or give the child a cool bath.

Should you consult the doctor?
Yes, it is important to consult the doctor for appropriate and prompt treatment of the underlying cause of itching.

What might the doctor do?
The doctor will examine the child and determine the cause of itching. She may prescribe anti-allergic/anti-histamine liquid/tablets and cream to be used locally to alleviate the symptoms.

If the child is unable to sleep because of intense itching and scratching, then the doctor may prescribe a mild sedative.

What can be done to help?
Keep the child's nails short to prevent him/her from breaking the skin when scratching. Use non-irritant cotton underwear for the child. Try and determine if a change of washing powder, fabric conditioner, or bubble bath may have caused itching. Keep calm and be reassuring.

Jaundice

This is yellowish discolouration of the skin and the whites of the eyes. It is a significant symptom of an underlying disease. The yellowish colour is due to the presence/accumulation of a bile pigment, bilirubin, in the blood. Normally bile pigment is made during the breakdown of old red blood cells and is disposed of by the liver. However, in certain conditions/illnesses there is an accumulation of the pigment in the blood causing yellowish discolouration of the skin. It may be accompanied by dark brown urine. In addition, the stools may be pale because of the absence of the pigment in the stools.

Is it serious?
Jaundice should always be treated seriously as it is a symptom of an underlying disease. It is less serious in newborn babies as it affects nearly one third of babies during the first week of their life. It is then called 'physiological jaundice' which is a normal phenomenon and usually no treatment is required.

What are the symptoms?
+ Yellowish discolouration of the skin and the whites of the eyes
+ Dark brown/red urine
+ Pale stools
+ Nausea, loss of appetite
+ Feeling unwell, fever, headache and weakness

What should you do first?
Get parents to consult the doctor immediately.
Give the child plenty of fluids to drink to prevent dehydration.
Be careful and meticulous about hygiene by scrupulous hand washing and boiling food utensils. This is particularly important if the child is found to have hepatitis.

Should you consult a doctor?
Yes, you should consult your doctor immediately.

What might the doctor do?
The doctor will carry out an examination and will determine the cause of jaundice. The child may be sent to the hospital for further tests and treatment as necessary. Depending on the cause, the child may be followed up at the hospital out-patient clinic until the problem is completely resolved.
If the child is found to have hepatitis, they will need to be isolated.

What can be done to help?
Follow the doctor's advice regarding any special diets and treatment. Try to be supportive and sympathetic. The child may feel tired, miserable and sometimes depressed for some weeks.

Measles

Measles is a common infectious disease of childhood which is now fortunately rare because of a national immunisation programme. It is a viral infection with a characteristic rash, fever and symptoms of a common cold or upper respiratory tract infection.

Is it serious?
It is usually not serious but the child may feel miserable and unwell. In some cases it can lead to serious complications, especially in children with chronic lung or heart disease and depressed immune system.

Is it infectious/contagious?
It is highly contagious.

What are the symptoms?
The incubation period is usually 10-14 days.
The symptoms are:
+ fever, which may go up to 40°C (104°F)
+ runny nose
+ dry cough
+ red watering eyes
+ rash appears 3-4 days after the first sign of illness. Initially, there are fine separate spots which coalesce giving a blotchy appearance. The rash appears first on the face, behind the ears and then spreads to the whole body. Tiny white spots with a red base (Koplik's spots) may be seen on the insides of the cheeks as the first indication of measles after the symptoms of fever and runny nose appear.
The rash starts to fade 3-4 days after its appearance and at the same time fever begins to subside. In the majority of cases the rash disappears within a week.

Are there any complications?
In some cases the child may develop otitis media (infection of the middle ear - see page 25) and pneumonia (infection of the lungs). In 1 in 1000 cases of measles, the child may develop the serious complication, encephalitis (inflammation of the brain by spread of infection to the brain or by an abnormal immune response to the measles virus).

What should you do first?
If the child has a temperature, keep the temperature down and ask parents to give paracetamol. Give the child plenty of fluids.

Should the child be excluded from nursery?
Yes, the infectious period lasts for about 5 days after the onset of the rash. The child should be kept at home and away from anyone else who may be at risk of infection. There is no need to keep the child away from siblings as the child is infectious before the rash appears and therefore very often the siblings have already been infected before the diagnosis is made.

Should you consult a doctor?
Yes, as soon as possible so that he can confirm the diagnosis. If the child gets worse and develops any of the following symptoms: earache, drowsiness, seizures, headache, vomiting, very rapid breathing, consult your doctor immediately.

What might the doctor do?
The doctor will examine the child and confirm the diagnosis. If the child has otitis media or pneumonia, he will be prescribed an antibiotic. If the doctor suspects that the child has encephalitis, the child will be admitted to hospital for observation and further treatment as appropriate.

What can be done to help?
Keep the child comfortable. Give him paracetamol to keep his temperature down* and plenty of fluids. Other children who have missed or have not had their measles vaccine are strongly advised to get immunised. MMR (vaccine against measles, mumps and rubella) is recommended around 13 months of age.

What is the outlook?
Most children recover completely within 10 days of developing measles. There is usually lifelong immunity against measles after a single attack.

*See *Administering medicine* page 5

Meningitis

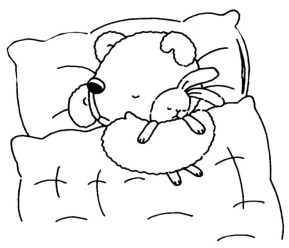

Meningitis is an inflammation of the meninges, the membranes covering the brain and spinal cord. It results from an infection with bacteria or viruses. A number of viruses may cause meningitis. Although bacterial meningitis is a very serious illness, it is still uncommon.

Is it serious?
Viral meningitis is not a serious illness and occurs frequently after mumps and in children over five years of age. However, bacterial meningitis can be life threatening or may lead to brain damage in some cases. With prompt diagnosis and treatment with antibiotics it can be treated successfully with a complete recovery. Bacterial meningitis commonly affects children under five, although it can occur at any age.

What are the symptoms?
In infants and younger children symptoms may be non-specific in the early stages, as follows:
✚ fever, can be high
✚ vomiting
✚ reluctance or refusal to feed
✚ irritability, increased crying or restlessness
✚ drowsiness

In addition there may be:
✚ bulging fontanelle
✚ inability to tolerate bright light
✚ generalised increase in muscle tone as rigidity
✚ red purple rash as fine, pinpoint spots spreading rapidly to the whole body, spots do not fade on pressure.
   THIS IS A VERY SERIOUS SYMPTOM AND REQUIRES IMMEDIATE MEDICAL ATTENTION AND TREATMENT.

In older children:
The symptoms may be more specific such as stiff neck due to increased rigidity of muscles, severe headache, and other symptoms as described above.

In some children:
✚ increasing drowsiness
✚ loss of consciousness
✚ fits

Most commonly, meningitis in children is meningococcal meningitis. These bacteria are normally found in the nose and throat and usually cause no symptoms. Another form of meningitis (haemophilus influenzae) has now become rare since the introduction of vaccine (HIB vaccine) which is given with other routine immunisations in babies. The causes of viral meningitis include mumps, influenza, chicken pox and glandular fever.

Should you consult the doctor?
If you suspect meningitis or if a child is unwell with any of the above symptoms, consult the doctor immediately, or take the child to the nearest accident and emergency department.

What might the doctor do?
The child will be admitted to the hospital and may undergo a lumbar puncture to confirm the diagnosis. This involves taking a sample of the spinal fluid by inserting a needle into the lower spinal cord. This is sent for laboratory examination.

In cases of rash and suspected bacterial meningitis, the child may be given high doses of antibiotics before he is referred to hospital or immediately on arrival at the hospital. Blood tests may also be done on admission. The child will be observed closely.

There is no specific treatment for viral meningitis other than symptomatic treatment.

For bacterial meningitis, high doses of antibiotics will be given for a period of 7 to 14 days depending on the nature of the organism. In addition, the child may require anti-convulsant drugs if they are irritable or having fits, and intravenous fluids and drugs to bring fever down. Close contacts of the affected children will be given antibiotics to prevent the spread of bacterial meningitis.

What is the outlook?
Viral meningitis usually leads to no long-term effects/complications. In cases of bacterial meningitis, early diagnosis and prompt treatment with antibiotics usually leads to complete recovery. In rare cases, in spite of early treatment, it may prove fatal.

The long-term effects of bacterial meningitis include seizures, delayed development leading to learning difficulties, deafness, spasticity.

Can meningitis be prevented?
Not all types of meningitis are preventable. Meningitis due to haemophilus influenza bacterium can be prevented by routine immunisation of babies (HIB vaccine).
One type of meningococcal meningitis (type c) can be prevented in short term by vaccine. The close contacts of the affected child are given antibiotics for 48 hours to prevent the spread.
In a situation where there has been more than one case in a school, the decision to vaccinate other pupils may be taken by the public health department. The programme is then carried out in conjunction with the department of community child health.

More advice and information is available from:

The National Meningitis Trust,
Fern House,
Bath Road,
Stroud,
Gloucestershire
GL5 3TJ.

Tel: 01453 768000.
The Trust also has a 24-hour support line: 0845 6000 800

Mumps

Mumps is an acute mild viral infectious disease of childhood. It has now become rare since the introduction of routine immunisation (MMR vaccine against mumps, measles and rubella) in childhood. It commonly affects children over two years of age. It has an incubation period of 14-21 days. Mumps affects one or both of the salivary (parotid) glands, which are situated in front of and below the ears and the angle of the jaw.

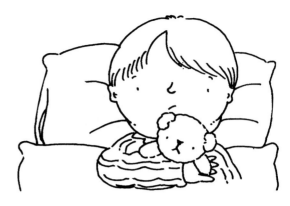

It is a notifiable disease in the UK. A single attack of mumps usually gives lifelong immunity.

What are the symptoms?
The striking feature may be the swelling of the parotid glands, which can be painful particularly on swallowing. In addition, the child may have:
+ fever
+ dry mouth
+ headache

Less commonly:
+ swollen and painful testes called orchitis
+ lower abdominal pain in girls due to swelling of the ovaries.

The swelling of glands occurs 1-2 days after the onset of fever and usually lasts for 4-8 days.

Is it serious?
It is usually a mild illness. In rare cases it causes meningitis or encephalitis.

Should you consult a doctor?
Consult a doctor to confirm the diagnosis. Consult immediately if the child has a severe headache, stiffness of neck, pain in abdomen or in the testes.

What might the doctor do?
The doctor will examine the child and confirm the diagnosis. There is no specific treatment for mumps.

If the doctor suspects that a child has meningitis or encephalitis, the child will be admitted to the hospital for further tests and observation.

What can be done to help?
Keep the child's fever down by giving him paracetamol* to reduce fever and relieve pain. Make sure that they drink plenty of fluids. Food may need to be soft and liquidised as the child may experience difficulty in swallowing.

Are there any complications?
+ Inflammation of the testes, called orchitis, occasionally in adolescent boys. Usually develops about a week after the onset of the parotid swelling.
+ Rarely encephalitis or meningitis.
+ Pancreatitis (inflammation of the pancreas) in some cases.

What is the outlook?
It is usually a self-limiting illness with full recovery in about 10 days.

Orchitis (inflammation of the testes) and pancreatitis usually do not have long-term effects. There is no evidence to suggest that orchitis leads to infertility.

Encephalitis or meningitis can lead to permanent hearing loss - either unilateral or bilateral.

*See *Administering medicine* page 5

Molluscum contagiosum

Molluscum contagiosum is a mild viral infection manifesting as tiny, white shiny papules (a solid circumscribed elevation of skin) on the skin, mainly on the face, hands, trunk and rarely on palms and soles. It is common in pre-school children but also affects older children.

The incubation period is 2-8 weeks. It is easily spread by direct or indirect contact, for example by touching or using infected towels or clothes and indirectly in a swimming pool or bath.

What are the symptoms?
The papules are discrete, pearly white, shiny in appearance varying in size from 1mm - 5mm, occurring mainly on the face, neck, hands, trunk, thighs and rarely on the palms or soles. The papules have a central dimple from which cheesy material can be expressed. There are no other symptoms.

Should you consult a doctor?
You should consult the doctor to confirm the diagnosis. It is usually a self-limiting condition, lasting a few weeks to a few months, although sometimes it can persist for years.

In some cases it will need treatment. This could be by piercing the papules/pimples with an instrument dipped in podophyllin paint, by scraping them off with a curette or by freezing them - but over-treatment may lead to scarring. Usually reassurance is required that it is a self-limiting condition.

What is the outlook?
Usually complete recovery within a few weeks to few months with no long-term effects. The child should keep his towel separately to prevent spread to other children and family members. It is important to treat children who also have eczema or immune deficiency to prevent rapid spread of infection and hundreds of lesions.

Otitis media

This is the infection and/or inflammation of the middle ear which occurs as a complication of upper respiratory tract infection, such as common cold, tonsillitis or pharyngitis.

The tube connecting the throat and middle ear, called the eustachian tube, is relatively short in children, therefore making them more susceptible to otitis media. The bacteria or viruses can easily spread to the middle ear from the throat. The tube can also be blocked by the enlarged and inflamed adenoids and lead to the build-up of secretions in the middle ear. This causes pain and can also lead to perforation of the ear drum.

Sometimes, the secretions can become thick, sticky and glue-like. It is difficult for this to drain away and can lead to the impairment of hearing - a condition commonly known as glue ear.

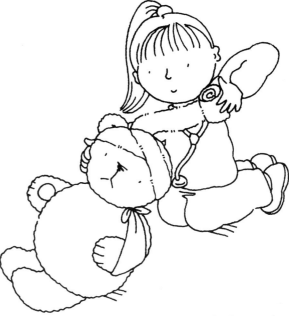

What are the symptoms?
+ earache
+ fever and vomiting in very young children
+ crying and irritability due to pain
+ not sleeping well
+ pulling or rubbing the ear
+ hearing impairment
+ discharging ear due to perforated ear drum

Is it serious?
It is painful and serious. It can lead to permanent loss of hearing if left untreated.

What can be done to help?
If a child has otitis media, they should see a doctor within 24 hours. Meanwhile, paracetamol can be given to relieve pain and fever*.

In older children, a well wrapped-up hot-water bottle against the ear with the child sitting up and the head turned downwards may also relieve the pain.

What might the doctor do?
The doctor will examine the child with an auriscope (an instrument to see the inside of the ear). If there is a discharge, a swab may be taken and sent to the laboratory to identify the germ. The doctor may prescribe an oral antibiotic. They may also check the child's hearing two to three months later. If a child gets recurrent middle ear infections their doctor may refer them to an ENT (ear, nose and throat) surgeon for further assessment.

What is the outlook?
Otitis media is more common in younger children up to the ages of seven to eight years old. After that the eustachian tube increases in width, enabling the fluid to drain easily. This reduces the frequency of middle ear infections.

*See *Administering medicine* page 5

- -

Rashes

Skin rashes are very common in children. They can be a symptom of a local or general infection or an allergy.

Common rashes in childhood are:
+ viral infection
+ roseola infantum
+ rubella or German measles
+ chicken pox
+ scarlet fever
+ molluscum contagiosum
+ less commonly, meningococcal infection

If there are no other symptoms or signs that the child is unwell, rashes are unlikely to be serious. If there is any doubt and if the child is very itchy or unwell, you should consult a doctor immediately.

Danger signs - seek medical help immediately
+ swelling of face or mouth
+ noisy or difficult breathing
+ difficulty in swallowing
+ purpuric rash (pin point spots which do not blanch on pressure)
+ increasing drowsiness
+ shock

What might the doctor do?
She will examine the child and make a diagnosis so that the appropriate treatment and/or reassurance can be offered.

What is the outlook?
Most rashes settle without any intervention. In others it will depend on the cause of the rash.

What can be done?
You should avoid any known allergens that may have caused concerns in the past.

Scabies

Scabies is not uncommon. It can affect anyone irrespective of social class and does not reflect lack of personal hygiene. It is highly contagious. It presents as an extremely itchy, irritating skin rash caused by a tiny parasite mite. The female mite burrows into the skin and lays its eggs - particularly in the clefts between the fingers, causing severe itching. Scabies is passed to another person by direct contact or from bedding which is infected with the mites.

What are the symptoms?

These may take up to six weeks to appear following infestation.
+ Intense itchiness, especially at night.
+ Fine grey lines (mite burrows) ending in a black spot, most commonly between the fingers but may also be found in the wrists, in the arm pits, between the buttocks, over the shoulders, around the genitals, on the palms and the soles.
+ Sores, blisters and scabs as a result of scratching.

Should you consult a doctor?

The child should be taken to see their doctor as soon as possible so that it can be treated promptly.

What might the doctor do?

The doctor will prescribe a lotion which kills scabies mites. The lotion is applied to the whole body except the head or neck. It is left for 24 hours and then washed off. It may need to be repeated in a day or two. The doctor may prescribe an ointment for intense itching. The whole family will need to be treated even if they do not have the signs of scabies.

The mites usually die within 3-4 days of treatment, although itchiness may persist for up to two weeks.

What can be done to help?

+ All clothes and bed linen should be washed.
+ All contacts of the child should be told that there is a risk of scabies so they can be examined and treated as appropriate.

Should the child be excluded from nursery?

+ The child should be kept away from nursery or school until after the treatment has been completed.

Scarlet fever

The introduction of antibiotics has made this now one of the less common of infectious childhood diseases. It is caused by toxins produced by a fairly widespread bacterium, streptococcus - the same bacterium which causes tonsillitis. The child has a scarlet appearance as a result of a generalised rash, hence the name - scarlet fever.

What are the symptoms?

The incubation period is usually 2-5 days.

The symptoms are:

+ Sore throat
+ Fever - which can be quite high (up to 40°C/104°F)
+ Vomiting
+ Headaches
+ Rash - starting on the chest and neck, appearing within 12 hours of first symptoms, small red spots merging together, spreading rapidly to the whole body (spots may be slightly raised). Rash lasts for 5-6 days following which the skin may begin to peel.
+ Flushed cheeks with pallor round mouth.
+ Tongue - initially thick white coating then changing to 'strawberry' tongue as red spots come up.

Are there any complications?

Scarlet fever is rarely serious. It can lead to inflammation of the kidneys (glomerulonephritis) and the joints and heart (rheumatic fever). With the use of antibiotics these complications are rare.

Should you consult a doctor?

You should consult your doctor as soon as possible if you suspect scarlet fever. You should consult your doctor at once if the child's urine is pink or smoky - suggestive of glomerulonephritis.

What might the doctor do?

The doctor will examine the child and confirm the diagnosis. A throat swab may be taken to grow the bacterium. Antibiotic treatment will be given for 10 days.

What can be done to help?

+ Keep the child away from other children until the course of antibiotics is finished.
+ Give paracetamol to reduce fever and relieve pain.*
+ Give the child plenty of fluids and a soft diet.

What is the outlook?

A single attack of scarlet fever gives lifelong immunity.

The child usually feels better within a week or so. If you are concerned that the child is not back to his or her normal self, ask parents to consult their doctor to rule out any complications.

*See *Administering medicine* page 5

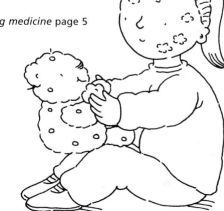

Spots   See 'Rashes' (page 25)

Temperature   See 'Fever' (page 16)

Urticaria

Urticaria (commonly known as nettle rash or hives) is a form of skin rash as a result of an allergic response or reaction - possibly to a drug (penicillin or aspirin) or certain foods (strawberries, milk, shellfish). It may also result from an insect sting or from direct contact with some plants. It is an extremely itchy rash presenting as smooth raised white lumps on a red base - known as weals. In addition, there may be swelling on the face.

Urticaria may be acute, lasting for 30 minutes to one hour. In some cases it may persist for several months. It may recur.

Urticaria may affect a small area of the body or it may be widespread.

Is it serious?
Usually it is not serious. However, it can be a part of severe anaphylactic reaction causing difficulty in breathing, difficulty in swallowing and abnormal drowsiness. **When this happens, it is an emergency and medical help must be sought immediately.**

Should you consult a doctor?
Yes. The doctor will ascertain the cause, if possible. In cases of severe anaphylactic reaction urgent medical help and advice must be sought.

What might the doctor do?
The doctor may prescribe antihistamine to be taken orally. It is also available over the counter at a chemist.

The doctor may give an injection of adrenalin if urticaria is part of a severe reaction.

In cases of chronic and recurrent urticaria, the child may be given oral corticosteroids and be referred to a dermatologist.

What is the outlook?
As the child gets older, the attacks of urticaria will possibly diminish.

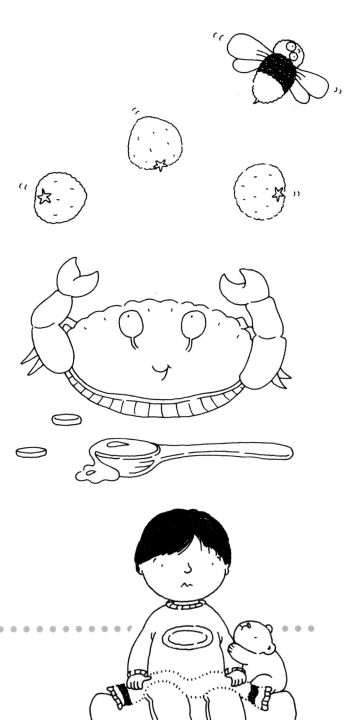

Vomiting

Vomiting is a symptom that all is not well. A single episode of vomiting in a well child is unlikely to be due to a serious illness.

Repeated vomiting may indicate the following:

+ infection of the gut, for example gastro-enteritis
+ obstruction in the gut
+ infection anywhere else in the body, for example ear infection, urinary tract infection, viral infection, meningitis
+ food poisoning
+ head injury

Is it serious?
If untreated it can lead to dehydration, especially in younger children.

What are the danger signs?
+ greenish yellow vomit
+ abdominal pain over six hours
+ flat, pink or purple spots which do not blanch on pressure

Other symptoms which may concern you:
+ abnormal drowsiness
+ vomiting for more than 12 hours
+ sunken eyes
+ dry tongue
+ not passed urine for six hours
+ not keen to drink any fluids

Should you consult a doctor?
Yes, if the child continues to vomit over a six-hour period.

What might the doctor do?
The doctor will assess the child and treat accordingly. The child may be sent to hospital for observation and intravenous therapy if necessary. She may prescribe an oral rehydration solution.

What can be done to help?
+ give the child plenty of fluids
+ check the child's temperature and give liquid paracetamol;* if appropriate.

What is the outlook?
It is generally good but depends on the cause of vomiting.

*See *Administering medicine* page 5

Warts

Warts are small, harmless, raised lumps or growths on the skin. They are caused by a virus and are contagious. They can appear singly or in clusters, most commonly on hands and feet but other parts of the body - such as face and genitalia - can also be affected.

Verrucae are warts which appear on the soles of the feet. Common warts tend to occur on the hands, feet and face. They are firm, raised growths with a rough surface. Plane warts are smooth, slightly raised and can be mildly itchy. They also occur on the hands or face.

Are they contagious?
Yes. They are usually by direct contact with an infected person.

Are they serious?
They are not serious or usually painful. However, verrucae can be excruciatingly painful. Most warts disappear within a few months but some may take up to a year to disappear spontaneously. It usually takes a couple of years for the body to build up resistance against the wart virus.

What can be done to help?
If you think a child has a wart, bring it to the attention of their parents and ask them to contact their doctor. Usually warts will disappear of their own accord. However, if they are causing discomfort or embarrassment, they can be removed by using the home treatments available for warts from the chemist. The manufacturer's instructions should be followed very carefully. Do not attempt to treat the warts on the mouth, face or genitalia.

Warts on the hands and feet are an easy source to infect others. Picking or scratching off the warts should be discouraged.

Verrucae and plane warts are treated by using a special plaster (salicylic acid plaster) and should be changed daily. Usually the treatment is effective in three weeks.

In other cases wart paint may be used (available over the counter) by following the instructions very carefully.

Should you consult a doctor?
The doctor should be consulted if you are unsure whether they are warts and the home treatment is unsuccessful. Facial and genital warts will need more specialist treatment such as freezing (cryotherrapy) or surgical removal.

What is the outlook?
Most warts usually disappear in months or years. But they can be a nuisance and therefore in some cases need further assessment and treatment.

• •

Wetting (nocturnal enuresis)

Bedwetting is more common than it is realised. Most children achieve bladder control at night by the age of three to four years. Twenty per cent of four-year-olds continue to wet the bed. However, the age at which children become dry is variable. Bedwetting is not a serious problem but it is frustrating for parents and carers.

Bedwetting may be:
+ primary - when the child has never achieved bladder control after the age when it is expected
+ secondary - when the child starts wetting the bed after a period of being dry (usually 6-12 months).

It is usually due to:
+ delayed maturation of the nervous system which controls the bladder
+ stress factors between the ages of two to four years
+ genetic factors
+ psychological factors

and uncommonly due to
+ physical factors, such as a urinary tract infection or an abnormality of the urinary tract. If accompanied by an increased thirst and frequency of passing urine this may be due to diabetes.

What can be done to help?
The child could be helped to get into a routine to pass urine regularly during the daytime and before going to bed. Make sure that the mattress is protected by a rubber sheet and covered by a top sheet which can be washed easily. The child should not be punished or humiliated for wetting the bed. This can be counter productive. He should be encouraged and praised when he is dry. A star chart may help some children to improve their motivation and give them encouragement and support.

In some children (aged over six and seven) an enuresis alarm (a pad and buzzer) may be successful. This device has a detector (a pad) which can be placed under the sheet or inside the child's pants. This is connected to a buzzer, which is activated when the child passes urine. This wakes up the child - who can take himself to the toilet. After a few weeks of being dry, the alarm can be discontinued. If unsuccessful, it can be tried again once the child is older and better prepared and motivated.

Parents should be helped to look at the stress factors at home and how they can be lessened where possible. A better understanding of this problem helps them to successfully manage this problem.

Should the doctor be consulted?
Yes, so that the child can be fully assessed. An explanation could be offered to parents and a programme started with parents to help their child. The doctor is also able to exclude a urinary tract infection or other physical cause and offer an appropriate treatment.

What is the outlook?
+ It is benign and self-limiting.
+ In most cases reassurance and support is all that is needed.
+ Most children stop bedwetting without treatment.
+ Older children may take longer to improve - enlisting a psychologist's help is useful in some cases.

Wheezing

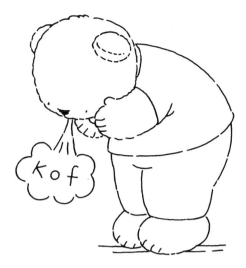

Wheezing is a common symptom in childhood - it is a whistling sound produced due to the narrowing of the airway. In the young child it is due to the swelling of the lining of the airway and the increased secretions causing the narrowing. In older children, in addition, there is a spasm of the smooth muscles lining the airway. In the majority of cases wheezing signifies asthma.

In a small number of cases it may be as a result of:
+ anaphylactic reaction
+ brochiolitis - acute viral infection due to RSV (respiratory syncytial virus) in young babies
+ foreign body
+ cystic fibrosis
+ obstruction inside the chest (mediastinum)
+ other infections such as tuberculosis

Whooping cough (also known as pertussis)

Whooping cough is a serious childhood illness with potentially severe complications caused by a bacterium called *bordetella pertussis*. It can be particularly dangerous in young children under one year of age. It is now uncommon in Western countries because of immunisation programmes. It is important to remember that it is an infectious disease which is preventable.

The incubation period is 7-14 days. It starts as a cold with a runny nose (catarrhal phase) which lasts for 7-14 days followed by a paroxysmal (spasmodic) phase for 4-6 weeks. Recovery usually takes another 2-6 weeks.

Period of infectivity - 7 days after exposure to whooping cough to 21 days after the onset of paroxysmal cough. The child should be excluded from the nursery during this period. The antibiotic Erythromycin may help to shorten the period of infection and is therefore recommended as a prophylaxis (preventive measure) to infant contacts.

What are the symptoms?

Initially:
+ runny nose, fever, aches and pains - usual symptoms of a common cold
+ a short dry cough, usually at night

Later on (after 7 days):
+ more prolonged coughing during day and night
+ excessive coughing with a sharp in-drawing of breath - producing a 'whoop' (in babies there may not be a 'whoop')
+ vomiting following a coughing episode
+ rarely seizures due to lack of oxygen to the brain as a result of prolonged coughing bouts
+ restlessness
+ chest problems due to collapse of a segment of the lung due to thick mucus causing a blockage of a breathing tube (bronchus)

What are the complications?
+ pneumonia
+ convulsions/seizures
+ episodes of apnoea (cessation of breathing)
+ permanent lung damage - bronchiectasis (rare)

Should you consult a doctor?
The younger the child, the more urgent it is to consult a doctor if you suspect whooping cough.

What might the doctor do?
The doctor will confirm the diagnosis. A sample from the back of the child's throat may be collected and sent to the laboratory for confirmation.

The doctor may prescribe a course of antibiotics for the child and close child contacts. Antibiotics are effective only if given in the early stages. If the coughing is severe with recurrent bouts of apnoea or possible seizures, the child will need to be admitted to hospital for nursing care, which may include oxygen, suction and tube feeding. The treatment of complications will also be needed as appropriate.

What can be done to help?
Keep the child calm, particularly during coughing episodes, gently stroking or patting their back. Simple physiotherapy may be helpful to clear chest secretions. This will be shown to parents. The child should not be left on their own in the bedroom. Give plenty of fluids to prevent dehydration due to vomiting. Give soft food to avoid vomiting.

What is the outlook?
Coughing may continue for weeks to months after the attack. Secondary infection may occur, for example pneumonia. Rarely, permanent lung damage may ensue. It is best to prevent whooping cough by ensuring that the child is vaccinated in the first few months of life.

Worms

There are a number of worms that can live in the intestines of human beings. However, in temperate climates threadworms (pinworms) are the most commonly found worms - primarily affecting children. They are highly infectious.

How is the infection caused?

The worm enters the body as eggs in contaminated food. These then hatch into adults in the intestine in 15-30 days. The female worm comes out of the anus at night to lay eggs around the anus. If the child scratches himself, he can easily pick up eggs in his nails and put them in his mouth without realising and start the whole cycle again. Threadworms are very small, white, thread-like, and only a few millimetres long (usually 2-12 mm). They are not easily visible unless you are looking for them.

What are the symptoms?

+ Itching around the anus, especially at night when the female worm lays eggs
+ Itching and redness of vulva in girls
+ Redness and inflammation of anus due to intense itching
+ Sometimes white thread-like worms seen wriggling in faeces

Should the doctor be consulted?

Yes, it is important not only to treat the child but the whole family. Rarely, the doctor may ask to collect eggs for microscopic examination. Eggs may be collected by pressing a piece of sticky tape on the child's anal region. This should be done first thing in the morning before the child uses the toilet or before they are washed.

What might the doctor do?

The doctor will prescribe the appropriate drug treatment which will paralyse the worm and will be passed in the stool. Treatment is usually taken as two doses 15 days apart. The doctor will ask parents to be meticulous about handwashing and general hygiene.

Is it serious?

No, it is not serious. It can be easily treated.

Other types of worms are:
Roundworms - these are rare in temperate climate but nevertheless children can be affected worldwide. Infection is most common in pre-school and young children. Roundworms are 10-15 cm (4-6 inches) long. Eggs are usually oval with a thick shell. Eggs are passed in faeces of infected individuals and mature in 5-10 days to become infective. Eggs are swallowed with contaminated food or water. Eggs hatch in intestines and are passed in faeces.

What are the symptoms?

+ Failure to thrive/under nourished (Be aware of roundworms if the child has recently travelled to an area where roundworms are common.)
+ Long worms in the stools.

Useful addresses

Association of Advisers for the Under-Eights and their Families (AAUEF)
c/o Maureen Norton
50 Whitehorns Way, Drayton
Abingdon, Oxon
Tel: 01235 531579

ACE (Advisory Centre for Education)
1b Aberdeen Studios
22 Highbury Grove, London N5 2EA
Tel: 0171 354 8321

British Red Cross
9 Grosvenor Crescent, London SW1X 7BR
Tel: 0171 201 5039

Council for Awards in Children's Care and Education (CACHE)
8 Chequer Street, St Albans
Hertfordshire AL1 3XZ
Tel: 01727 847636

Child Accident Prevention Trust
4th Floor, Clerks Court
18-20 Farringdon Lane, London EC1R 3AU
Tel: 0171 608 3828

Department of Health
Richmond House, 79 Whitehall
London SW1A 2NS
Tel: 0171 210 3000

Health Education Authority,
Trevelyan House, 30 Great Peter Street
London SW1P 2HW
(Useful for guidance on immunisation)
Tel: 0171 413 1976 (immunisation team)

Health and Safety Executive HQ
St Hughes House, Stanley Precinct
Bootle, Merseyside, L20 3QY
Tel: 0151 951 4000

National Childminding Association (NCMA)
8 Masons Hill, Bromley, Kent BR2 9EY
Tel: 0181 464 6164

National Children's Bureau
8 Wakley Street, London EC1V 7QE
Tel: 0171 843 6000

National Society for the Prevention of Cruelty to Children
42 Curtain Road, London EC2A 3NH
Tel: 0171 825 2500

Playgroup Network
PO Box 23, Whitley Bay
Tyne and Wear, NE26 3DB
Tel: 0191 252 1516

Pre-School Learning Alliance (PLA)
69 Kings Cross Road, London WC1X 9LL
Tel: 0171 833 0991

Professional Association of Nursery Nurses (PANN)
2 St James' Court, Friar Gate, Derby DE1 1BT
Tel: 01332 372337

RoSPA Royal Society for the Prevention of Accidents
Edgbaston Park, 353 Bristol Road
Birmingham B5 7ST
Tel: 0121 248 2000

St Andrew's Ambulance Association
St Andrew's House, 48 Milton Stret
Glasgow G4 OHR
Tel: 0141 3324031

St John Ambulance
1 Grosvenor Crescent, London SW1X 7EF
Tel: 0171 235 5231

Child information form

Name of nursery/pre-school: _____

Child's full name: _____ Date of birth: _____

Parent/Guardian name: _____

Address: _____

_____

_____ Postcode: _____

_____

Emergency contact names:

1 Name _____

Address _____

_____ Tel no _____

2 Name _____

Address _____

_____ Tel no _____

3 Name _____

Address _____

_____ Tel no _____

(Please write in order of priority, ie who you would like us to contact first)

Family doctor: _____

Name: _____

Address: _____

_____

Tel no: _____

Medical details/conditions

Does your child have any medical conditions we need to know about? Any allergies or special dietary needs?

_____

_____

_____

Signed (Parent) _____ Date _____

PRINT NAME _____

Signed _____ Date _____
(on behalf of nursery)

PHOTOCOPIABLE

Accident/incident form

(to be completed for all accidents and illnesses occurring on the premises or during any activities managed by the setting)

Nursery/pre-school worker in charge:

Job title:

(please tick appropriate box)   **Illness** ( )   **Accident** ( )   **Near miss** ( )

Name of child injured or ill

Description of symptoms/injury

General description of treatment *(if administered)*

Result

Name of person evaluating or treating

Description of incident

Time of incident   **Date of incident**

Parent / carer informed Name

(please tick appropriate box)   **By letter** ( )   **phone call** ( )   **in person** ( )

Parent's/carer's response/comments

Is there any indication that they will be taking further action on any matters?

Action taken to prevent a recurrence

Name of person completing form

Signature   **Date**   **Time**

Reported and logged according to HSE regulations:

Signed   **Date**